What others are saying about working with Erin Tumas.

"In 'Mind Over Fatter' Erin is addressing the single most important issue when it comes to weight loss and health; the inner game, how your thoughts and beliefs determine the results you get. Erin has learned from her own experience and from some of the best teachers in the world. If you are a person who is not getting the results you want or has a history of not getting results that last, Erin's approach will help you."

Robert MacPhee
Director of Training, The Canfield Training Group
Author, "Manifesting for Non-Gurus"

"Erin is a game changer in the health & wellness field! Instead of the same old concepts that don't work and just create more dependency and frustration for people, Erin teaches foundational, core principles that will absolutely shift your awareness, perspective and attitude toward your body and how your health supports your life's mission. Powerful!"

Sean Smith, Master Results Coach
Moorpark, California

"Erin is a skilled and gifted storyteller who willingly shares her own story, all the while inspiring and offering tips on the "how to's" of beginning and pursuing our own journey. Do read this book. She has a powerful message for YOU!"

Lila Larson
President Coaching Links, Inc, Winnipeg, Canada

"Erin will inspire you to be your best self – body and soul. You will learn to balance goals with healthy and practical steps ultimately achieving optimal health and an inspired life."

Stephanie Perez
Mother of two, Laguna Beach, CA

Mind Over Fatter:
The Secret to Thinking Yourself Thin

Copyright © 2010 Erin Tullius

ISBN 978-1-60910-449-8

All rights reserved. No part of this publication may be reproduced, stored in a retrieval system, or transmitted in any form or by any means, electronic, mechanical, recording or otherwise, without the prior written permission of the author.

Printed in the United States of America.

Erin Tullius
A Paige by Paige Publication
www.MindOverFatterBook.com
2010

DISCLAIMER

The purpose of this book is to educate and entertain and may not be construed as medical advice. The information is not intended to replace medical advice offered by physicians. The author and/or publisher do not guarantee that anyone following these techniques, suggestions, tips, ideas, or strategies will become successful. The author and/or publisher shall have neither liability nor responsibility to anyone with respect to any loss or damage caused, or alleged to be caused, directly or indirectly by the information contained in this book.

Mind Over Fatter:
The Secret to Thinking Yourself Thin

Erin Tullius

For further information and support visit:

www.MindOverFatterBook.com

Learn about:

Upcoming FREE Teleseminars

Upcoming *Mind Over Fatter* workshops

Free downloadable products

Mind Over Fatter fitness camps

And MUCH more!

This book is dedicated to my beautiful boy, Tyler Shea, who remains my greatest teacher.

Acknowledgments

To my teacher, Jack Canfield, who gave me the courage and inspiration to actually put pen to paper and complete this book. For that I am truly grateful.

Thank you to my wonderfully supportive family for always believing in me. I would especially like to acknowledge Mike for his editing help, to my dad for listening to hours of content on the phone, and to my husband Steve for encouraging me to sit and write (and for the gentle pushes when I needed them!) Thank you to my mom, Piper, Virginia and the Tullius family for the interest they took in this project.

For my girls Ami and Natalie who have taught me what a true "girlfriend" is, I am eternally grateful.

Thank you to my 2009/2010 Train the Trainer family who inspire me to be great. You have given me wings.

Lastly, thank you to the men and women who trusted me with their health and fitness programs throughout the years. You are the reason I wrote this book. It is because of your questions I learned that until one changes their mindset, the "tools" will never make it out of the toolbox.

I love and appreciate you all.

Table of Contents

My Story 1
Chapter One: Dispensable You? 7
Chapter Two: Hold Yourself Accountable 13
Chapter Three: It's Not In Your Jeans! 21
Chapter Four: Is Serving Food, Serving You? Or Living
    with Purpose 27
Chapter Five: Your Thoughts, Your Health 35
Chapter Six: Take it to the Limit 41
Chapter Seven: Letting Go 47
Chapter Eight: Shutting Up the Self-Talk 53
Chapter Nine: Go for the Goal! 59
Chapter Ten: Motivated or Inspired? 65
Chapter Eleven: Someone to Watch Over Me 69
Chapter Twelve: Cavemen Did It 73
Chapter Thirteen: Conscious Consumers 79
Chapter Fourteen: You Like to Move It! 85
Chapter Fifteen: Committed 89
Chapter Sixteen: Falling Off the Treadmill 93
Chapter Seventeen: Oh, What Fun! 97
Epilogue 101
Mind Over Fatter Recommended Resources 103
About the Author 107

My Story

Much of my teenage years were spent as the girl on the cheerleading squad who was a little heavier than the rest. I don't know that I would have been described as fat (though you never know with teenagers), but I was definitely heavier than the other girls and I knew it. Sure, I was a cheerleader, but every time I donned the navy and white uniform I worried someone might laugh. It might also be crucial to mention that I happened to live in the Mecca of incredibly beautiful, insanely wealthy, and perfectly un-plump teens also known as Newport Beach, CA.

Despite my abhorrent eating habits, college was actually much kinder to me with my weight struggles. I'm not sure if it was the cafeteria's fine cuisine, the distance from my "comforting" father, the penny pinching meals, the copious amounts of liquid courage, or just the fact that I frequented the school's gym. It was probably a mix of everything (except for maybe the alcohol). I was down to a size 8 and feeling pretty good.

After college, I stepped up the workouts a notch (though I kept up the partying and fast food) and maintained a relatively fit size 8. After a long series of events, I eventually ended up living with my fiancé, jobless and depressed. I turned to my longtime comfort: food and simultaneously stopped the workouts. I got a job working 70-80 hours a week on an incredibly measly salary, worked tirelessly to plan my own wedding, and I felt physically awful. I continued to gain weight.

A week after the wedding, my new husband and I moved several hours away to start his business as a chiropractor. Prior to the move, I decided to pursue my love of Pilates and got certified to teach. The previous chiropractor had a small rehab facility that I eventually turned into a small Pilates studio. Working 70-80 hours seemed like a breeze compared to owning our own business, but at least what we worked for was ours. Months went by and I continued to gain weight. Along with the weight gain, I was in a constant fog and chronically exhausted. Doctors told me I was just "depressed", but I knew there was more to the story. I had historically been more of an optimist and this new depressed state felt more like a symptom of the other symptoms that plagued me rather than the catalyst.

As it turned out, the stress from my whirlwind year (and several years before that!) had wreaked havoc on my adrenal glands and thanks to a Naturopathic Doctor, I started taking an adrenal supplement. My fog lifted, I had the energy to work out again, and I eventually got back to my usual size 8.

About a year later, just after a Christmas party, I peed on a stick and it said "Pregnant." What?! I had just gotten my body back to "normal" and I was starting to actually feel pretty good. Pregnancy was a whole new ballgame.

For those of you who have never been pregnant, I have to tell you that while some women feel the "glow" of their unborn child in their womb, I just felt like a constipated, beached whale with some massive hormones. My son decided to arrive on his own time, which happened to be very late. I clearly recall stepping on the scale at my last appointment when my midwife exclaimed, "Wow, you're just shy of 200!"

Did I hear her right? Two-hundred what? My bowling score? Surely she didn't mean 200 pounds!! I left the office in frustrated, pregnant lady tears.

After my son's birth, I had secretly hoped he was at least 10 pounds and that at least another 40 was just water. Well, 7 pounds 14 ounces and about a week later, I stepped again on the dreaded scale and realized my worst fear. I was still 185 pounds. I went back to teaching

Mind Over Fatter: The Secret to Thinking Yourself Thin

a Mommy and Me class on my son's 6-week birthday and I thought for sure I was going to die. I was short of breath, my arms and legs quivered, and I thought I might drop my son right in front of the class (all 10 pounds of him). I couldn't believe how out of shape I felt. As I drove away, I cried again. This time they were frustrated, post-partum tears.

By the time my son was 18 months, after what seemed like an endless and extremely arduous process, I was back into my size 8s. But something felt different. As I began to fit into my old favorite clothes and buy new ones, I began to realize that 8 was definitely not enough.

I had enjoyed studying the personal development masters since I picked up Anthony Robbins *Unlimited Power* at the ripe old age of 21. I was familiar with the power of affirmations and positive self-talk. For the first time in my life, I looked at my size 8 body and began to see my "self" as a smaller size.

It was then that I was reminded of the story of Roger Bannister. In the 1950's, there were several men who had attempted to run one mile in less than four minutes. After numerous unsuccessful attempts, it was thought to be impossible. Some runners came extremely close; however, it seemed that 4:02 was the best that was humanly possible.

On May 6, 1954, however, all that changed. That day, at a race in Oxford, Bannister ran the mile in 3:59.4. That day was historic for one main reason: it was now possible to run a mile in less than four minutes.

A mere 46 days later, the record was beaten. In fact, since that day, the record has been beaten several times. Bannister, though the first one to break the time barrier, actually held the record for the shortest amount of time. Once he proved it was humanly possible, it became easier for others to follow his lead.

Though my revelation was not world-record breaking, it was certainly a breakthrough. I was going to do what had never seemed humanly possible. I began to tell myself, "I am so happy and grateful now that I am a size 6" each morning as I got dressed. I focused mainly on the feelings I would feel if that were, in fact true. As I had never been a size 6 in my adult life, there was a certain amount of detachment from the outcome that I had not felt previously. It was more of a "Wouldn't it be nice to be a size 6..." rather than "I must, I must..."

A mere 6 weeks after I began this regimen, I headed to my favorite store for a few new summer clothes. As I sifted through the racks, I found myself pulling size 8s to take to the dressing room. When I asked for help with a few things, the sales woman said, "OK, what are you? A 4 or a 6?" I laughed out loud. I grabbed the 8 and high tailed it for the dressing room. And then something magical happened.

I put on the first pair of adorable, size 8 capri pants. Too big. "They must run large," I thought. I pulled on another pair, and another...all too big. Could it really be that simple? I walked out of that store a size 6.

Now, don't get me wrong; I do not claim my transformation was solely the result of my affirmation. There was some nutrition, exercise, and portion control involved, but I now saw my goal as something that was actually possible. So possible, in fact, that I did it again and became a size 4!

I wrote this book so that you too might make a new realization about yourself, about your health, and about what is possible for you. With anything, there will be things that challenge you, but there will also be things that make you feel like you just won the lottery. I will tell you things that may be difficult for you to hear, but I promise that they come from a place of love. I will be your coach and your friend, but I will also give you a push when you are in need of one. You deserve success, you deserve to be healthy, but most of all, you deserve to be happy.

With Love & Gratitude~

Erin Tullius

Chapter One:
Dispensable You?

"Take care of your body. It's the only place you have to live."
Jim Rohn

We live in a society where "quick and easy" is the mantra. Almost everything seems to be dispensable, disposable, or at best, recyclable. So our world is filled with paper plates, paper shopping bags, e-waste, old cars, disposable diapers, disposable this and dispensable that.

It is no wonder that we treat our body as if it is disposable too! The messages in our media state, "If you get too fat, just get the lap band!", "If you're too ugly, we can fix that, too!", "Heck, you didn't really *need* that body part anyway!" and if you are still hesitant, "We can give you a new and improved (insert body part here)!" But let's take an honest look at where this mentality has gotten us.

Our need for more dispensable things has put us in our current economic situation, has made humans (by far) the sickest species on the planet, has put our one and only planet in a state of crisis, and has given us a big pile of crap (pardon my French) in return.

You, my friend, are not dispensable! You are given one physical body that is supposed to last for your 120 years. That body is your vehicle to fulfill your purpose and there are many people on this planet who are in need of things that only you can provide.

When you fill your body with greasy hamburgers, alcohol, caffeine, cigarettes, toxic cleaners, pesticides, antibiotics, drugs, soda, etc. and do not give it the things it needs (fruit, veggies, water, protein, sunlight, etc.) it will die before your spark does. This is not meant to be harsh or cruel, but merely to cause you to think of the gravity of those seemingly minor decisions. No amount of medical intervention can keep you alive if you do not do the things necessary for your survival. The human body was created with a perfection that is so beyond our comprehension we can only begin to understand the minute, yet vital workings of it.

Think of your most valued possession...something that means the world to you. Think of that wedding gown, car, antique, piece of jewelry, etc. How would you feel if someone poured alcohol on it, blew cigarette smoke on it, surgically removed a piece of it, poured toxic chemicals on it...you get the picture. So why is it ok to do this to our bodies? Why do we deplore this type of behavior when it comes to our "valued" possessions and not when we do it to the one thing that truly belongs to us alone?

When you strip it down, (pun intended) your body is the only thing you've got left. Everything and everyone else is just extra.

Once at a seminar, we were advised to list the top ten things we truly felt we were passionate about. We were then asked to narrow it down to just three. While I pondered which things to prioritize, two great realizations came. The first was that most of the activities I enjoyed were things that weren't possible if I wasn't in good physical condition and the second was that keeping my body healthy was not something anyone else could do for me. As Jim Rohn put it so succinctly, "You can't hire someone to do your push-ups for you."

You see, no matter how much you love spending time with your family or working in a field you love, none of those things will matter if you are unhealthy. When you do not take the time for health, you will be forced to make the time for sickness. Personally, I'd rather take the former.

Mind Over Fatter: The Secret to Thinking Yourself Thin

What good is nature if you can't go explore it? What fun is a game if you can't join in? How much interaction can you have with your kids if you don't have the energy? How good can your relationships be if you are always focused on how bad you feel? How can you be productive in business if your brain feels foggy?

Life cannot be experienced to the fullest if our bodies are not fully functioning. You have heard doctors say things like, "Well, your blood pressure is normal, your cholesterol is low and you have a pulse. You are perfectly healthy." But are you really?

Let's imagine Dr. Freeman is going over his patient, Mrs. Jones' paperwork. He sees that the nurses have taken her blood pressure, her pulse is normal, and all of her vital signs are within normal range. Dr. Freeman sees all of these and determines that Mrs. Jones is ready to be discharged from the hospital. It is then that the nurse turns to Dr. Freeman and says, "But, doctor, Mrs. Jones is in a coma." Mrs. Jones may have her vital signs, but she certainly doesn't have quality of life!

Are you merely your vital signs? Your vital signs may be able to give you markers for certain disease (though even that is debatable); however, they can tell you little about your quality of life. If your vitals are normal but you are constantly fatigued, are you living life to the fullest? If your vitals are normal, yet you are 50 pounds overweight and not able to play on the floor with your kids, are you living life to the fullest? Of course not. We all want to play at 100%.

As a fitness expert, I have been approached by people looking for tools to help them accomplish their ideal physical body. I would work really diligently to get them all the information they needed for their nutritional needs by reading countless books and spending hours researching. I developed exercise programs and gave stress-reducing tips. Much of this was to no avail. Why? The common thread was that there was something going on in their psyche that was preventing them from achieving their goals. In many cases, they may not have had clearly defined their goals or set any goals at all. Others had limiting beliefs about their weight or their available time or how their financial situation affected them. Regardless of the issues, the tools they needed were not only the nutrition information or the exercise routine. They needed to know how to make lasting lifestyle changes when it came to their beliefs about themselves.

A lifestyle change is something you decide to do for the rest of your life because you want to, not because you have to lose 50 pounds or get your cholesterol in check.

When Bob Bedford decided he was ready to make some changes, he weighed a whopping 512 pounds. He described himself as your average Joe with a wife, two kids, and a job that was maybe slightly more stressful than usual. He worried that he might never see his little girls get married or even graduate high school. In an instant, he made the decision to change. He contacted his doctor and said he did not want surgery. He wanted to get fit the "old-fashioned way."

Bob began to eat right and hit the gym daily and in only 2 ½ years, he lost 257 pounds! That's the size of a refrigerator and the weight of two people! But Bob was determined to survive to see his girls grow up. He took that determination and did not waiver in his quest to become healthy.

Bob may seem like an extraordinary person, but just like anyone else, he set a goal, and he accomplished it. He was committed to sharing his life with the family he loved. We all have that motivation within us.

This book will take you through a series of question-and-answer processes to assist you in finding your inspiration and accomplishing your physical health goals. You may even find that these tools are useful to you not only in your physical goals, but also in many other areas of your life.

Mind Over Fatter: The Secret to Thinking Yourself Thin

It may help you to have a pen handy as some of the processes will require writing. You can either write inside the book or on a separate pad of paper. You may want to read one chapter at a time and implement it, or read the whole thing through once and then go back. It is entirely up to you. While picking up this book was an excellent first step, the success lies in the implementation of the book rather than the reading of it. Your outcomes will be a direct result of the extent to which you implement these ideas.

I applaud you on your path to treat your body as the indispensable thing it is. The good news is you have already taken the most difficult step! Let's get the ball rolling and find your inspiration!

Chapter One Lessons:

- You are not dispensable!
- No amount of medical intervention can keep you alive if you do not do the things necessary for your survival.
- You can't hire someone to do your push-ups for you.
- Vital signs do not indicate a life of vitality.

Chapter One Affirmation:

"My body is my most valued possession. Without it, my spirit would be without a home. Everything I do depends upon the existence and vitality of my physical body and I appreciate each and every intricate piece of it."

Chapter Two:
Hold Yourself Accountable

Often, when we find ourselves in an undesirable situation, we immediately find someone to blame, we look for excuses, we complain, or we justify our actions. But what does that do for us? How do you feel when you blame, complain, make an excuse or justify?

When it comes to health, the most common excuses are related to lack of time, lack of money, or lack of energy. If these sound familiar, let's delve a little deeper.

We all have the same amount of time in any given day, correct? You have 24 hours and so does every other living thing on the planet. Can you think of someone who seems to be really busy, but is also very physically active? Is there someone you know who seems more successful than you in business or with their family, AND works out daily? If your answer is yes, you can see that it is possible. If it is possible for them, then it is also possible for you and everyone else.

How many hours a day are you spending watching T.V.? Be honest. The average American watches 6 hours a day. If you simply cut out one hour of T.V., you will find your time to work out or prepare healthy meals.

How much time do you spend aimlessly searching the internet or watching YouTube videos?

How often are you sleeping in simply because you don't "feel like" getting out of bed?

Are you starting to realize where you might have more time?

Let's take a look at the "lack of money" excuse. How much food do you spend money on that you know is not healthy (Starbucks, ice cream, fast food, etc.)? Do you have cable? Buy nice clothing? Drive an expensive car? Go on several vacations? Maybe none of the above is true for you, however, do you own a pair of running shoes, have access to a body of water to swim in, own a bike, or have a T.V. where you could play a DVD? Hmmm...get the idea?

Lack of energy can be a major obstacle because it is one of those vicious cycles we get caught up in. First, you must ask where your lack of energy is originating. Have you allowed yourself to gain more weight than your body is comfortable handling? Do you have a physical issue that you have chosen to use as an obstacle or excuse? Is your diet high in sugar, carbohydrates, or dairy? Have you researched different nutritional philosophies to find out why you may be experiencing a dip in energy?

You see, the more you continue to make excuses about why you are not getting fit, the further you begin to spiral and allow yourself to remain stuck. **What if you made the decision today to hold yourself 100% accountable for everything in your life?** What might you be doing differently?

Life comprises a series of happenings or events. It is impossible to predict everything that may or may not happen. It is, however, up to you to choose your response to those events.

It is easy to get caught up in the negativity and emotion that follows events such as the Haiti earthquake or JFK's assassination. You were not directly responsible for those events, but there are many who allow themselves to be overcome with sadness or pain even if they had no direct connection to the event. Having compassion does not mean compromising your soul to do so.

Mind Over Fatter: The Secret to Thinking Yourself Thin

You see, if you allow yourself to become consumed by grief, sadness, anger, or fear, you rob the world of your gifts. If you decide to let your emotion stop you from being healthy, you are not able to give what you are here to give and we all suffer because of it.

By making yourself accountable, the excuses begin to disappear and you will start to understand that in order to bring the world your gifts, your health is vital.

If the idea of 100% accountability is a bit too much to bear right off the bat, **What if you were to take 5% more responsibility for your health?** Would you start taking vitamins, join a gym, walk 20 minutes a day, or eat less fast food? Begin now by making the commitment to 5% more and you may find that within a short while, it is that much easier to make the jump to 100%.

Tammy was in my coaching program and wanted to lose 100 pounds. It seemed as though every time she began to make any strides in a positive direction, she became injured. First it was her knee, then she developed debilitating cysts, a death in the family pulled her off track, and then it was a knee flare-up. After some time, I began to point her back to how she had been sabotaging her own progress by blaming the events in her life instead of taking responsibility. By taking just 5% more responsibility, she began to realize how she was attracting all these events in her life in order to keep herself overweight.

You see, there is always good reason for keeping things the way they are. When you were a child, do you remember a time you stayed home sick from school? You may not have felt well, but there was certainly a payoff. You were allowed to watch T.V., showered with attention, given whatever you wanted, and allowed to miss a day of school. Being sick might have been pretty fun.

What has been your payoff? Does not exercising leave you more time to work on your career or more time with your family? Does eating chicken wings and fries and drinking a beer on Sunday with the gang allow you to be more social? Does holding on to extra weight mean you don't have to be vulnerable to new relationships? I'll wait while you figure it out...

You are going to have to be really honest with yourself. Write it all down. What has been the benefit for staying unhealthy?

Once you are able to see how your situation has benefitted you, it becomes easier to let go of that belief that is no longer serving you. Most importantly, once you see how you have benefitted, you can take on more responsibility for your new actions.

Have you ever complained about the service at a restaurant to everyone at your table, but never approached the manager to see about improving it or simply decided to eat elsewhere? Have you ever complained about your spouse at work and then gone home to your spouse to complain about your co-workers? What about blaming fellow travelers for the long lines at the airport? How many times have you complained or blamed someone for something they had no power to change?

It's a funny little nuance about our culture. It seems that we are notorious for our complaints. If we would like to make a change, doesn't it just make sense to voice our concern to the people who may actually be able to help us?

Start holding yourself accountable for your complaining. When you complain, it means there is another outcome you were hoping for, but that you didn't want to risk getting it. Take the risk and ask for what you want or stop complaining about how you wish it could be. There is nothing wrong with either option as long as you take the time to realize that your complaining is not getting you anywhere.

My father loves to write. He also loves to complain. Several years ago, he was working as a handyman and he was miserable. It wasn't so much that he hated the handyman work; in fact, I think he rather enjoyed it. He was not pursuing his passion however, and at the end of the day, he was miserable because he had not had the time or energy to do what he really loved, which was writing.

One day, I had heard enough of his complaining and I told him that I refused to listen to it anymore. He either had to complain to someone who could do something about it, stop calling me, or stop doing the handyman work. Thankfully, for everyone involved, he chose the third option and he has been all the happier since.

When it comes to your health, where are you complaining? Is it too cold to work out? Too hot? Do you need better shoes? A gym membership? Need to lose weight before you step foot in a gym? What is it?

Stop your complaining and begin to take action. Let's face it, nobody ever got in shape by sitting on the couch thinking about why they couldn't. Stop saying why you can't and start thinking about how you can.

How long does it take to change your actions or beliefs and make a new decision? A day, a week, a month, a year? If you started to change your actions or beliefs today, how long would it take until it was changed? There are time parameters placed on everything these days. It takes 30 days to create a habit. It takes 90 days to double your income. But, how long does it take to make a change?

If you decide today that you would like to be a singer, when is it that you become one? You become a singer in the moment you decide you are one. And how long does it take to decide? An instant, a moment, a second!

You can make the decision today that you are health-conscious; you are someone who loves to run, a physically active person, someone who eats mindfully. Of course, there is always room for improvement, but it only takes a moment to decide that you already are what you want to be. Once you make the decision to go down that path, it makes no difference if you have been doing it for years or mere moments. You make the choice. When it comes to your health, nobody can make that choice for you.

You are 100% responsible beginning now. Act as if everything is happening because of you, not to you. I guarantee you will begin to see things in a new light. Let go of the complaining and blaming. These types of things only mean you are not willing to make a change.

What would the world be like if Gandhi simply sat back and complained about the injustice occurring in India? What if Martin Luther King, Jr. had blamed others for their attitudes towards the African American people instead of taking action? It was their ability to recognize where the world wasn't working and their inspiration to change it that made a difference. Whether you agree with them or like them or not, their actions changed the world.

Each action has a ripple effect. What or whom will your actions with regard to your health affect? Did your father die young from heart failure due to an unhealthy diet? Did your mother live a long and fulfilling life because she chose to always eat healthfully? Would you say that the choices of your parents affected you regardless of whether you decided to mimic those actions? Whether or not you realize it today, your actions have already begun to ripple. What do you want that ripple to look like? It is up to you and you alone.

You are 100% responsible beginning now. Not tomorrow or someday in the future. Tomorrow is always in the future. Tomorrow is always tomorrow. What about today? When would now be the time? Now!

Chapter Two Lessons:

- ➢ By making yourself 100% accountable, the excuses begin to disappear and you will start to understand that in order to bring the world your gifts, your health is vital.

- ➢ Begin today by taking 5% more responsibility for your health.

- ➢ Nobody ever got in shape by sitting on the couch thinking about why they couldn't.

- ➢ It takes only an instant to make the change.

Chapter Two Affirmation:

"Today I choose to be 100% accountable for my life and my action or inaction. It takes only an instant to make the decision to take 5% more responsibility for my health and fitness. From this moment forward, I will make life happen rather than allowing life to happen to me."

Chapter Three:
It's Not In Your Jeans!

You mean my butt? Well, maybe that is what's in your jeans, but we're talking more than Levi's or Sevens, people. We are talking those tiny little buggers that we all like to blame for our problems. Our genes.

One of the most common excuses people make for being overweight, out of shape, or simply unhealthy is that they have a family history of poor health, obesity, overweight, etc. With the new biology of *epigenetics*, this idea no longer holds water. BUT...this is GREAT NEWS!

Yes, we are given a set of genes from birth. No, we cannot change our genes. Yes, there are a very small number of genetic diseases or disorders (such as Down's syndrome). However, we CAN change the way our genes express themselves!

Our genes are like little light bulbs. We have several of them throughout our houses and we can turn them on and off at our leisure. If I make the choice to drink a diet soda with aspartame (a known carcinogen) every day, I may switch on my cancer gene. So...is it because I have the gene that I got cancer? NO!!! It's because I engaged in behavior that flipped that cancer gene switch.

The genes nearly always express themselves in response to their environment. Each time a gene expresses, it switches on or off just like a light bulb that we control with the switch. If I want to stop expressing my cancer gene, or prevent my system from doing so, I need only stop flipping the switch. Sometimes it takes a long time to get the switch to turn on, and sometimes it takes a long time to turn off. Sometimes, the bulb may burn out before you can get the switch to turn back off. Sometimes too many switches have been flipped and it becomes an issue of trying to figure out exactly how to switch them off or on again. No matter the case, it is ever so important to know that it is possible to change the expression of your genes.

Now, sometimes our lights go out because the electric company has an outage. Unfortunately, no matter how many times we try to flip that switch, the lights won't go back on until we change our environment. Take the people living in Hinkley during the Erin Brockovich and PG&E debacle. Those people could have been doing everything right when it came to their health. It would not matter one bit, because the water they drank, bathed in, cooked with, etc. was filled with extremely toxic chemicals. Their environment was killing them.

So, what choices did they have? If we stick with the light bulb analogy, they could buy a generator to turn them back on (begin a series of treatments independent of their environment such as living in a holistic center for 30 days), they could go somewhere that had power (move), or they could choose to live independently from any power company and run their homes on solar (drink and bathe in potable water from another source). The point is they did have a choice to change how their genes were expressing themselves.

So, why do I see so many people who are overweight and came from a family with overweight parents?

It's primarily because they have developed the same habitual patterns. They eat the same foods, live in the same area, have the same sleeping habits, the same thought patterns, etc. Those habitual patterns that have been ingrained either consciously or subconsciously are causing the genes to express themselves in either a positive or a negative way.

Even when great distance divides families and children are grown, there are certain belief patterns that have been created. Children will often follow in their parents footsteps, but in some cases, two health nuts may create an extremely resistant child if the information is presented in a way that makes the child feel they have no freedom of choice.

Food as reward is also a pattern that is becoming more and more common. Candy and junk food are inexpensive and can easily pacify or comfort a child. It's not that taking your kids for ice cream after a job well done is detrimental; however, I would encourage parents to think about other rewards that might be healthier for both themselves and their children.

What about things like cancer or diabetes?

Again, as difficult as this is to hear, these are diseases of lifestyle. This might be difficult to swallow because nobody wants to believe that their actions caused their cancer or their child's diabetes. Most often, we can look at diet. Also, those that worry about getting cancer or diabetes because their family members have had it tend to become ill with the same diseases. Why? Just as discussed above, there are certain patterns that our family has ingrained; however, this is largely the work of our powerful minds. What we focus on we bring into being…that goes for positive and negative.

Our society has become so focused upon finding a cure that we have forgotten about prevention. Detection and diagnostics are not prevention. What I mean is that by getting a mammogram, you are not actively preventing breast cancer; you are checking to see if you already have it. No amount of checking will stave it off.

To a large degree, we have come to accept that once we have a disease, we must take medication to correct the damage. I am not recommending should you have a disease, that you stop taking your medication. I am recommending that you take this as a wake-up call to change your diet and exercise habits as well. As long as you continue to poison your body with the things that made it sick in the first place, you will remain ill. The body is a remarkable self-healing organism and will work its magic when you give it the fuel it needs to do so.

Chapter Three Lessons:

- Dr. Bruce Lipton and the science of epigenetics state that our genes, though passed down from our parents, are largely controlled by our environment.

- Our genes can be thought of as light bulbs which we can turn on and off when we change our environment.

- Habitual patterns that have been ingrained either consciously or subconsciously are causing our genes to express themselves in either a positive or a negative way.

- Detection and diagnostics are not prevention.

Chapter Three Affirmation:

"Though I have been given a set of genes, I have the power to control my environment and therefore, to change the expression of my genes. I no longer subscribe to a defeatist mentality when it comes to my health and well-being. I actively seek wellness."

Chapter Four:
Is Serving Food, Serving You?
Or
Living with Purpose

What is your life purpose? What are you here to accomplish? What makes you feel fulfilled? Have you ever even stopped to think about it?

Whether you are completely unsure or just a tad unclear, a life purpose can help you define what is best for you and your health.

When I met Sue she was a wonderful, beautiful, intelligent woman (she still is!). She had defined her life purpose and was pretty well on track in most areas of her life. At that time, she wanted to be a personal development trainer more than anything. Her life purpose was clearly to educate and inspire others. Sue had one major problem. She didn't feel inspiring. She didn't feel comfortable in her own skin at 50 pounds overweight.

When she approached me to help her "lose weight," I asked her how her current weight was limiting her. She shared her lack of confidence in getting in front of a group and I asked her about her life's purpose. Poor thing had no idea what was in store for her when she asked for my help!

We began by doing a trust fall from the stage at an event we were both attending. After several agonizing minutes of sobbing and terror, Sue did the trust fall. She was open to trusting and I began to work with her.

I asked her to think about everything she was doing to her physical body as if it would either assist her in her life's purpose or detract from her achieving it. How would this extra piece of bread help her or harm her? How would sleeping late help her or harm her? How would choosing the elevator versus the stairs help her or harm her?

Sue began to see that each and every thing she did could be run through the filter called her "Life Purpose."

Sue was attending a workshop and was asked to go to dinner with someone whom she had connected with over the previous days. She was in a quandary over what to do because she had decided to do a meal replacement shake program and that particular evening was supposed to be a "shake" evening. She chose to go to dinner and beat herself up about it for several days thereafter.

I asked her to then run that evening through her life purpose filter. As she did, she realized that in that particular moment, the dinner was more critical to her purpose than the shake. And guess what? That's OK! It's not that the "healthier" option will be the winner, but it certainly will win out much more often.

So, what is your life purpose? There are numerous methods and trainings to assist you in the formation and discovery of your life purpose. I have devised the following exercise to give you an idea.

If you are using a separate piece of paper, divide your paper into 4 columns. Write one of the following words in each column: Purpose, Love, Strengths, and Important.

In the **Purpose** column, I want you to think about what it is you feel you were born to do. Think about those things you truly feel you are called to do. They don't need to be laser-specific. In fact, it may be better if they are a bit more generalized (i.e. to educate others, to connect humanity, to heal the planet). It is easy to get lost in the form that those actions take or in how we express those things and lose sight of the actual essence of our purpose.

Take a moment and write the top 5 things that come to mind when you think about your life purpose.

Purpose

1.

2.

3.

4.

5.

Next, let's look at what you **Love** to do. Again, try not to get lost in the form that this takes and get to the true essence of what it is you truly love to do.

Love

1.

2.

3.

4.

5.

Thirdly, we will look at your **Strengths**. These are qualities you consider strengths as well as activities in which you distinctively excel.

Strengths

1.

2.

3.

4.

5.

And lastly, think about those things that are **Important** to you. What is it that you value? What do you consider non-negotiable?

Important

1.

2.

3.

4.

5.

Go back over each of the above categories and circle the top 3 in each category. You may notice some common themes that begin to emerge. With this information, construct a sentence or two that feels inspiring to you. It may take some time or several drafts to revise; however, eventually you will find something that you can work with.

Rewrite your statement and put it anywhere you may look before you make a decision.

The refrigerator or pantry is a great place to start! The next time you go to reach for an extra cookie or a big bowl of ice cream, it may serve as a gentle reminder to take care of your body so that you may fulfill that purpose to its fullest.

Even before this, ask yourself if your kitchen is filled with healthy options or if you are setting yourself up for sabotage. If the answer is the latter, I suggest you simply open up the pantry and simply remove the junk from the house. Yes, it really is that simple. The next time you want ice cream at midnight, you may find it is much more difficult to track down if it isn't housed in your freezer.

At first, you may want to run each and every choice you make through your life purpose filter. Ask yourself, "Is this choice bringing me closer to or further away from my life purpose?" I will reiterate that the healthier option may not always win. The point is to start looking at life in a more purposeful, confident way.

Remember that the choices are up to you. You can decide to take yourself either closer to or away from your dreams. Which would you rather do?

Chapter Four Lessons:

- A life purpose can help you define what is best for you and your health.

- The PLSI (Purpose, Love, Strengths, Important) Exercise is designed to give you more clarity on your on life purpose.

- Set yourself up for success by clearing the house of food and distractions you know take you further from your goals.

- You can decide to take yourself either closer to or away from your dreams by using your life purpose as a filter in the decision-making process.

Chapter Four Affirmation:

"I am living a purpose-filled life and each of my decisions assists me in the fulfillment of that purpose. (Insert your own life purpose statement here.)"

Chapter Five:
Your Thoughts, Your Health

You may be wondering what your thoughts have to do with your health. You may be feeling as if your body is just different and that it is not possible for YOU to be fit and healthy. These feelings are merely your inner critic attempting to rationalize your current state of health and well-being. It is wholly within your power to change your current state of health. But...don't believe me. There are several other experts who have addressed topics such as the Law of Attraction and Quantum Physics, so this is by no means new information. It may, however, be new to you.

Though this is not the focus of this book, I think it is important to recognize and become familiar with these theories simply because it will help you to feel empowered.

Law of Attraction

The basic principle of the Law of Attraction is the idea that Like attracts Like. In this case, it is the idea that your thoughts will create a frequency or vibration that causes those thoughts to become reality. We have all heard of people who have had miraculous recoveries from some illness. Often we hear that these people have remained positive through their experience. The Law of Attraction theory would ascertain it was their thoughts of health combined with their healthy choices that created their recovery.

The Law of Attraction is also often called coincidence, serendipity, miraculous, fortuitous, answered prayers, and many other things. In reality, we are asking God, the Universe, Buddha, Allah, (or any other name you resonate with) for that which we want, we are taking the necessary inspired action, we receive that which we want, and we send our thoughts and emotions of love and gratitude in return.

When I first learned the basic theory, I began wishing and hoping that everything would just suddenly appear into my reality. When the car, the money, the friendship, or whatever else did not appear, I found myself diving into a state of doubt. I didn't realize that it wasn't just about wishing and hoping. I also needed to take action when I got an intuitive hit despite how loudly my mind told me to ignore it.

Just as I mentioned in my own story, it is important to release your attachment to the outcome. The harder I wished and hoped and pleaded with the Universe to provide, no matter how grateful I was for what I already had, the more resistance my mind created. When we approach our desires from a wishful point of view, we are introducing an element of doubt. What I mean is that the more you are hoping and praying, the more your mind thinks that there is a possibility it may not happen.

There are many fabulous resources for the Law of Attraction and I am not able to go into great detail, however, I do feel this is an important concept to familiarize yourself with. I have included several references in the "Reference" section of this book if you wish to delve deeper. You may prefer to look into the study of quantum physics if a more scientific approach resonates with you.

While you may or may not understand the concept in its entirety, I suggest you keep it in mind as you begin your journey to health and fitness.

Psychoneuroimmunology

A term coined by Dr. Robert Ader. Dr. Ader was experimenting with saccharin water and rats. He gave them the water combined with an injection that made them nauseous. That injection was also known to suppress the immune system. He then gave the same rats the saccharin water without the injection and the rats had the same reaction. In fact, many of the rats began to die.

Dr. Ader found that this was because the rats still experienced the same physical reaction in both experiments. Their bodies were unable to distinguish the saccharin water from the injection. As a result, the rats ended up with severely depleted immune systems and eventually became so easily susceptible to disease that they died.

Since that first experiment, psychoneuroimmunology has become a field of phenomenal study and research allowing many to realize the true power of the mind-body connection.

Visual Motor Rehearsal

Dr. Denis Waitley was the Chairman of Psychology for the U.S. Olympic Committee during the 1980's. He hooked the athletes up to sophisticated equipment and had them visualize competing in their event. Remarkably, the same muscles fired when they visualized as when they were physically participating in their sport. The brain was not able to distinguish a vividly imagined event from one that is actually occurring.

It is now widely understood in the Olympic world, the importance of visualizing your preferred outcome.

Dr. Bernie Siegel and Louise Hay

Dr. Bernie Siegel is a medical doctor who, while working with cancer patients, began to notice that one of the biggest factors in determining whether or not the patient survived often had more to do with their emotional state than their physical state. He started working with patients with all kinds of illnesses and has found this to be profoundly true for the broad spectrum of people who are ill.

Louise Hay has done work in the realm of emotions as the cause of the disease, and not merely part of the cure. She ascertains that every ailment can be traced back to not only a physical hurt, but an emotional one as well.

I bring the work of these two to light simply because if you do find yourself in a situation of less than perfect health, many people have found these to be valuable resources.

Chapter Five Lessons:

- It is wholly within your power to change your current state of health.

- It is important to recognize and become familiar with these theories simply because it will help you to feel empowered.

- Law of Attraction states that like attracts like. The theory states that our thoughts will create a frequency or vibration that causes those thoughts to become reality.

- Psychoneuroimmunology, visual motor rehearsal, and the work of experts such as Dr. Bernie Siegel and Louise Hay are fabulous resources to tap into and understand the power of the mind over our physical body.

Chapter Five Affirmation:

"My thoughts are powerful and attract the blessings of health and vitality as I open up to the power of universal energy. I remain in a state of love and gratitude and my body continues to gain health with each passing minute. I am grateful for my physical body and I choose today to attract the healthiest body possible."

Chapter Six:
Take it to the Limit

What is it that's holding you back? What beliefs or actions are you allowing to run you? I used to know a limiting character by the name of Needy Nellie. The following poem best describes Nellie and her journey:

Needy Nellie
Needy Nellie had a knack of reaching for a hand
Needing someone all the time
Someone to understand

She needed one to listen to
And one to listen back
She needed one to tell a joke
She needed teacher, Jack*

She needed one to shop with her
She needed one to call
She needed one to step out and do anything at all

And so through life she wandered
Needing someone all the while
Hoping that no matter what
Someone would make her smile

She was disappointed often
As the people in her world
Could not always be there when she needed them—poor girl

'Til one day Nellie woke up in the bed all by herself
Reaching for another's hand, her own was all she felt
Maybe if I ask it, my own hand will suffice
Will give me what I'm needing
Though a friend would sure be nice

So Needy Nellie grabbed her hand and brought both to her heart
Took in a breath of gratefulness then took those hands apart
She felt power, safety, happiness and lifted up her chin
It was then that Nellie realized all she needed was within.

*Refers to Jack Canfield, whom Erin studies with extensively.

If you haven't already guessed, Nellie was a lovely persona I chose to identify myself with when I was avoiding authenticity. If Nellie made a commitment to herself to go the gym and she didn't have a buddy, she might have decided to ditch the gym and go out for coffee with a friend. She may have had a wonderful time, but in the process, she would lose her commitment and trust in herself. She allowed her sense of neediness to distract her from what she wanted and if she continued to do so, she would never accomplish her goals.

Maybe Nellie is difficult for you to relate to, but what about Whirlwind Wanda, Baloney Bob, Play Small Paul, Meek Matilda, Hypochondriac Hilda or Unimportant Uma? We all have limiting characters that we allow ourselves to play for whatever reason. As I mentioned before, there is a payoff for keeping it the way it is, but what about the reward of making change?

Ask yourself what you are doing to limit your progress? How do you sabotage yourself? If you can't think of anything, ask some people you know well how they see you limiting yourself.

If you like, create a character that incorporates those limiting qualities and name him/her. When choosing a name, make sure to pick something that is in no way related to your own name. The goal is to dissociate from this character, and giving them your name may serve to bring the two of you closer together!

The bottom line is, write down a list of what it is that's limiting you from accomplishing the body and health of your dreams. Once you make these realizations, you'll be able to recognize when you are allowing them to limit you.

Nellie was a limiting character, but we also have limiting beliefs we allow to run us. A limiting belief is any belief based upon prior conditioning that limits your ability to perform or achieve your true passion. These beliefs may be either conscious or subconscious. They may be a result of things you were taught by parents, teachers, coaches, or peers. They may be the result of some negative self-talk which took place following an event. They may be a mantra you have heard in different societal applications. No matter where they come from, they do not serve you.

My limiting belief when it came to my weight was, "I'll never be a size 4. I'm just not built for it." For years, I carried that around…as a size 8. I honestly believed that no matter what I did, I would never fit into anything smaller than a size 8. One day, I decided to put myself to the test (keep in mind this is post-baby) and let go of this belief.

I created a new affirmation, "I am so happy and grateful now that I am a size 6." Within one or two months, with some effort, but not anything Herculean, I went to the store to buy a new outfit. The woman helping me asked, "What size are you…6? 4?" I laughed out loud. I took the size 8 back to the dressing room and was astonished at how large it seemed. I left that store a size 6.

At that point, I thought, "Well, if I am a size 6 now, it wouldn't be that much more difficult to try for a 4." I promptly changed my new affirmation to, "I am so happy and grateful now that I am a size 4."

And again, as if some genie had overheard my wish and granted it, I very quickly and seemingly effortlessly became a size 4.

What is it that you keep telling yourself to keep you in your current state?

"I had a baby and now I am always just going to be fat."

"My parents died young, so I will too."

"As long as I stay overweight, men will not approach me. If I don't play the game, I'll never have to lose."

"I have never been very coordinated and exercise just isn't for me."

"Being fit and healthy is too difficult, too expensive, too time-consuming, etc."

"I live to eat and I love food too much."

It makes no difference what the belief. Any of these beliefs can eventually sabotage progress you hope to make until you recognize them and just let them go.

Figure out what is limiting you, how it is limiting you, and simply let it go. It will not serve you on this journey. It is time to leave the bags behind and get on the plane. You will not need anything inside those bags once you reach your destination.

Chapter Six Lessons:

- Everyone has limiting beliefs. You are not alone.

- Once you make these realizations, you'll be able to recognize when you are allowing them to limit you.

- Create a new affirmation to solidify your commitment to letting go of your limiting belief.

- It is time to leave the bags behind and get on the plane. You will not need anything inside those bags once you reach your destination.

Chapter Six Affirmation:

"I choose to let go of my limitations and open up to the possibilities that lie within. I free myself from the constraints of these limiting beliefs and give myself permission to fully express myself."

Chapter Seven:
Letting Go

When I was a young girl, my parents would take me to play games at a little arcade near our home. I would play Skee-Ball and Whack-a-Mole in an effort to accumulate as many tickets as possible. More tickets equaled better prizes from the prize case. Being that these games were not my strongest suit, I usually ended up with some jacks, a bouncy ball, and a Chinese finger trap.

Have you ever seen a Chinese finger trap? If not, they are very simply a small cylindrical toy about 6 inches long. When you place two fingers inside and then try to pull them out, your fingers become stuck. I distinctly remember one particular time I stuck my fingers inside and they got immediately stuck. I began to panic and looked around for someone to help me remove them. Sensing my anxiety, my parents immediately obliged and pushed both ends of the trap together, setting my small fingers free.

The trick with the finger trap is that, in order to remove it and set yourself free, you must bring your fingers closer together.

Letting go is a lot like the finger trap. Often, we try to resist it. We frantically try to pull away, creating more and more tension. That tension creates more anxiety and the anxiety pulls us further and further away from our true essence. It is the idea that what we resist persists. In much the same way, we must embrace those emotions that are keeping us from accomplishing our ideal bodies, and our ideal lives. Once we learn to embrace our fears, insecurities, and doubts, we are then ok to let them go.

Excess weight is a funny thing. Sometimes we are so focused on letting go of the weight, we forget all of the other things that are waiting for us to let them go. Women who have been abused will often carry around their "shield" to protect them from getting hurt again. Men and women who feel insecure in themselves may carry around weight to help their subconscious "prove" that they are not loveable or that they are unattractive.

The secret is not in following the steps necessary to lose weight, but in the fact that if we let go of what is holding the weight on, it will let go of its hold on our bodies. As long as the emotion remains, the weight will too.

Also, the more we resist doing those things that we know are necessary, the more the negative situation will fester. If you are resistant to beginning an exercise regimen, for example, you may find your frustration level increases as you continually gain weight despite the fact that you have not changed any of your habits. What we resist most definitely persists.

Our subconscious mind loves us so much that it wants to make sure we are right all the time. So what does it do? Once we make a decision, no matter how ridiculous it may seem; our subconscious mind will find a way to prove that decision true. It is constantly searching for proof.

It's like the person who goes around proclaiming the world is out to get them. Sooner or later, the subconscious mind finds a way to make them think this is true. In no time, they lose their job, crash their car, and even get gum on their shoe…twice. All of these things then serve as proof that the world truly is out to get them!

This type of cyclical thinking will only make you miserable. Let it go!

Letting go, however, doesn't only refer to letting go of these deep-seated beliefs. It is also about letting go of attachment.

Mind Over Fatter: The Secret to Thinking Yourself Thin

Have you ever wanted something so badly that you would have sacrificed anything to get it…and then you didn't get it? I am sure we have all experienced this. When I was a young child, I wanted nothing more than to be an actress. I would dream all day about the types of roles I would play, the costumes I would wear, the boys I would kiss (oops! Did I write that out loud?!). I wanted it so badly, but I was so attached that dream that it didn't come about until much later. Until I let go of my attachment to the dream.

When you "want" or "need" something, you are acknowledging a place within you that feels lack. If you said you wanted a supermodel body, it implies that somewhere within, you don't believe it is possible. The more you want/need it, the less you believe in the possibility. Not only that, but the more you "want" something, the less grateful you begin to feel about what you currently have.

There is a huge difference between wanting or needing something and thinking, "Wouldn't it be nice if…"

It's not that you must take a blasé approach. In fact, the feelings associated with your desired outcome are crucial, however I have found the more you can let go of your attachment to the outcome, the easier it will come about.

This letting go process can become quite simple by focusing on appreciation. If it's thinner thighs you are looking for, appreciate your thighs and legs for holding your body upright, for transporting you around, for helping you hike, or jump, or play basketball. If it's a flat stomach you desire, appreciate your torso for holding all your organs in place, for carrying a baby, for digesting your food, for providing a place to rest your hands. Once you begin to appreciate your body for the great services it provides and let go of a need to have it be different, you may find your body transforms.

There are many releasing techniques which are truly wonderful, but I also know of a very simple way to let go. Something I call "releasing through your eyes", also known as crying. Have you cried lately? The body has a wonderful way of allowing us to release emotion through tears. Tears are completely natural and there is nothing wrong with crying.

Crying can be cathartic and refreshing to the body just as rain to the earth. Let your body release your emotion in the form of tears every so often.

Let's take a lesson from the Chinese finger trap, and embrace those things you find yourself resisting in order to get the results you are looking for.

Chapter Seven Lessons:

- Letting go is a lot like the Chinese finger trap.

- Once we learn to embrace our fears, insecurities, and doubts, we are then ok to let them go.

- Sometimes we are so focused on letting go of the weight, we forget all of the other things that are waiting for us to let them go.

- There are many releasing techniques which are truly wonderful. Several are listed in the resource section of this book.

- Let your body release your emotion in the form of tears every so often.

Chapter Seven Affirmation:

"I let go of the things and emotions that have been taking up space in my emotional bank. As I create space for new emotions, life suddenly becomes more effortless. When a new emotion arises, I allow it to be present, I embrace it and accept it, and then I let it go. The more I choose to let go, the lighter I begin to feel."

Chapter Eight:
Shutting Up the Self-Talk

Some researchers estimate that our self-talk is up to 80% negative and only 20% positive. Knowing what we have just learned about the impact of our thoughts on our reality, **WHY ARE WE LISTENING???**

Some people do not realize the power of this type of negative thinking. Others do not think there is anything they can do to change it, turn it off, turn it down, or shut it up! Still others do not realize just how often they are thinking negatively.

Typically, when our inner voice speaks, I believe it has one of three different tones or "voices." In order to shut those voices up when they are not assisting us, I have devised a method you may find helpful to be able to discern who is speaking.

The Inner Child

This is the voice that wants to scream and kick and throw a tantrum when you don't get your way. It is the one that puts others down in order to feel superior or makes snide remarks. This is also the voice that wonders how things work and why with a genuine curiosity, and the one that speaks of dreams and wishes. The inner child will let you know when it is time to leave work and go play. It will also let you know when you are taking things all too seriously.

It is important to listen to this voice when it is giving you useful feedback. For example, if it is telling you to go and play instead of spending Saturday on your computer, it may be a good idea to go play. If it's telling you to go play when you are in the middle of surgery, it's probably best to wait until the surgery is complete before you act on that instinct. It is, however, a possible indicator of your lack of trust that the surgery is the best thing for you.

Treat this voice as you would your own children. Nurture this voice when it speaks from wonder, joy, and genuine curiosity, and let it know when its comments are not appropriate. Also recognize that the inner child may be appropriate much more often than we give it credit. Play is vital! And heck, you just might be getting some exercise while you're playing!

The Inner Critic

We all know this one well. This voice may even sound a bit like your parents, your teachers, or some other authority figure. This voice may say things like, "You aren't good enough or smart enough to do, be or have that." This voice rarely has anything positive to say, or does it? If we relate this voice to the role of the parent, we can begin to see how this voice comes from a place of protection.

Imagine your small child runs into the street. You may yell at them, ask them what on earth they were thinking, and be very critical. Does your yelling mean you love them any less? Of course not.

That child may not fully understand what they have done to displease you. They may even be angry with you. You, however, only yelled and became upset because you love your child and understand that there can be fatal consequences to running in the street. What you failed to explain to the child was that you are not angry because they are "bad," but because you love them so much you couldn't stand the idea that they could be hurt or killed.

Your inner critic is the voice that protects you from harm, be it physical or emotional. This is an important voice to listen to if you are in a dark alley and some suspect characters begin to approach you.

It is also responsible for the chatter that happens when you have that "gut" feeling that someone is not being honest with you.

Your inner critic is designed to help you despite the nasty things it likes to say sometimes. Ask your inner critic why it is giving you the feedback and then discern whether or not it may be useful to you.

The Inner Coach

This third voice can be very motivational at times. This voice tells you how great you did in dance class or how proud of you it is. This voice, too, can have its dark side. It can be critical, angry, and downright mean. Your inner coach can also be a challenge in performance situations. If you have ever played a competitive sport, you may have had a coach like this. The inner coach is tough because it can see that there is something better available to you and it would like to see you living up to your potential.

I once had a cheerleading coach I wanted to strangle at times. If our routine wasn't perfect, we would do it until it was...even if that meant staying until 9:00 at night. We wore 3 pound ankle weights to make sure our jumps and kicks were as high as they could possibly be.

One evening in particular, a week or so before competition, our team was exhausted. We were all nursing badly bruised and battered bodies and it was already about 10 p.m. We thought we were performing the routine for the last time, and as the music finished, we heard the dreaded word, "Again." I think we all burst into tears. We had to dig deep and did it once more. Though I was not happy about the situation at the time, I knew our coach cared about us and she knew we had enormous potential. We placed 3rd out of about a hundred teams in that competition. I firmly believe it was because of the challenge of our coach that we were able to do so well. She was our biggest critic when she needed to be, but when we succeeded, she was also our biggest cheerleader.

Though our inner coach might push us a bit, it is because this voice knows how wonderful we truly are. Our coach always wants us to perform to the fullest extent of our potential. Your inner coach may sound disappointed at times, but remember it is only because it recognizes your greatness that it knows when you are choosing not to recognize your greatness. Just as with the other voices, try to discern what it is your coach is really trying to say and take whatever feedback may be helpful.

Living with 3 Voices

The Inner Child, Inner Critic, and Inner Coach are all useful voices. They speak to us in times of need. All these voices perform vital functions, so it may be unwise to shut them up entirely. The more you understand why they tell you the things they do, the easier it will be for you to know what is helpful and what is unnecessary.

I have not yet met anyone who did not hear these three voices and so I am willing to bet that they are present for us all. That means we must live with them. It does not mean we must let them run us.

We all have something else that I call your authentic self. Your authentic self is the "you" that listens to these three voices, or in some cases, talks back. The voices are not your authentic self. Your authentic self is the observer of the voices.

Quieting the Voices

The first step in quieting the voices when they are not useful is to simply recognize when they are speaking, thank them for their observations, and let them know that your authentic self will take it from there.

Many of us vacillate between two places called memory and fantasy. We live in either the past or the future. We look forward to, we fantasize, we remember, we dream, we recollect, but rarely do we just

Mind Over Fatter: The Secret to Thinking Yourself Thin

"be." When we live in the past (i.e., "I used to be a size 8...") or the future ("I really want to be a size 8..."), we have much to be critical of. In reality, it is only because we are living in the past or the future that we have these regrets.

Be comfortable with where you are today. It's ok to want to work towards something different, but celebrate the small steps you are currently taking. Forget about the cake you ate yesterday or the jeans you hope to fit into. Be where you are today, because that's the only place you can be. You are in the perfect place at the perfect time and your body is perfect today. It may be better tomorrow, but the only way you can make that happen is by making a different choice now.

The more present you find yourself, the more the voices will begin to quiet themselves. Remember, you can make the choices starting now.

Chapter Eight Lessons:

- When our inner voice speaks, I believe it has one of three different tones or "voices."

- Your inner child is the voice that wants to scream and kick and throw a tantrum when you don't get your way.

- Your inner critic comes from a place of protection.

- Your inner coach can be critical, angry, and downright mean or it can be a great source of motivation.

- Your authentic self is the "you" that listens to these three voices, or in some cases, talks back. The voices are not your authentic self. Your authentic self is the observer of the voices.

- The more present you find yourself, the more the voices will begin to quiet themselves.

Chapter Eight Affirmation:

"I thank my inner child, my inner critic, and my inner coach for their ability to protect me from harm, to motivate me to do my best, and to honor my desire to have fun. I appreciate the valuable feedback they have to offer. I choose to allow my authentic self to decipher when the voices are assisting me in my purpose and when they are merely detracting from it. My authentic self serves as my guide."

Chapter Nine:
Go for the Goal!

We all have goals, dreams, hopes, and wishes. I have yet to meet someone without something they hoped to accomplish during their time on this Earth. I have, however, met many people who do not strive for those goals, who think they are unrealistic, who are unclear on their goals, and who have given up on their goals.

Goals do not have to be any of those things. Goals do not have to be large or seemingly unattainable, they don't have to be depressing, and they don't have to be intimidating. A goal is simply a statement of something you want to do. It can be as simple as having a goal to go to the grocery store today or as seemingly complex as losing 100+ pounds. Either goal is just fine as long as it feels good for you.

If you do nothing else with this book, I would suggest you at least write out your health and fitness goals. Have you ever gotten in the car and not known exactly where you were going? Maybe you had a general idea of your destination, but you most likely took several wrong turns to get there. What if, however, you have GPS? It makes the journey a while lot easier.

Think of your goals as your GPS system. With a clear idea of where you are going, the path becomes much clearer. Why not make things easier on yourself, right?

There are a few guidelines for goals that may help you as you set out to write some. Goals must be clear, definable, attainable, and measurable in order to be truly effective. They must also be written down. Resist the temptation to push the goal further out or make the goal smaller in size because of any fears or roadblocks. A goal is about stretching yourself a bit. If it feels good, go with it!

The following are a few examples to assist you in writing your goals:

Clear

I want a new car.

Vs.

I want a new, pearl Ford Escape Hybrid with tan leather interior

Definable

I want to lose 10 pounds

Vs.

I want to weigh my ideal weight Of 140 lbs.

Attainable

I want to lose 20 pounds by Jan 2012 at 5 p.m.

Vs.

I want to weigh 180 pounds by this weekend

Measurable

I want to feel healthier

Vs.

I want to be able to chase my kids on the soccer field for at least 15 minutes

With the guidelines in mind, create at least one goal for each of the following timelines. It may help you to start with the end goal and work backward.

My Goals Sheet

What are the goals you wish to accomplish within the following timeframes?

3 months from today (Date:_____)

_____

_____

6 months from today (Date:_____)

_____

_____

1 year from today (Date:_____)

_____

_____

5 years from today (Date:_____)

_____

_____

Any other goals you wish to accomplish within a different timeframe:

_____

_____

_____

_____

_____

_____

Once you have solidified some goals, type them up or write them out several times and place them in prominent places around your house, your workplace, and/or your car. Make sure to read them over at least once each day so that you can keep yourself aligned with what it is you want. Your goals may shift and change over time, and that is ok. Just make a new goal and keep on going!

A Word of Caution:
In my experience, the biggest mistake I have seen is when one sets a goal and when the deadline approaches and it is not accomplished, the person beats themselves up over it. If the goal was to become a size 8, for example and you were a size 14, the fact that you are now a size 12 becomes completely irrelevant in your mind because you did not

accomplish your goal by the set deadline. Any progress is a success! Set a new goal and move on. You cannot change what is now, but you can change your future outcomes starting now.

Chapter Nine Lessons:

- Goals do not have to be large or seemingly unattainable, they don't have to be depressing, and they don't have to be intimidating. A goal is simply a statement of something you want to do.

- Goals must be clear, definable, attainable, and measurable in order to be truly effective.

- Make sure to read them over at least once each day so that you can keep yourself aligned with what it is you want.

- The biggest mistake you can make is to set a goal and then when the deadline comes and you have not accomplished it, you beat yourself up over it. Set a new goal and move on.

Chapter Nine Affirmation:

"The goals I set are clear, definable, attainable, and measurable and therefore, I effortlessly attain them. Each time I read my goals, I align myself with the vibration of accomplishment. My goals are within my grasp. I merely need to reach out and grab them!"

Chapter Ten:
Motivated or Inspired?

Imagine you are living in the savannah. You stoop down to take a drink of water from the river, and as you lift your head, you spy a tiger on the other side. His eyes are fixated upon your every move and you instantly realize you must find a way to get away quickly. Your adrenaline begins pumping as he takes a step closer and then, without thinking, you RUN!

Until the tiger finds a tastier option, you get away, or you become dinner, you are motivated to do one thing and one thing only. Once you find your house and successfully secure the doors, you take a deep breath and feel grateful for your survival. You begin to think about all the things you may not have accomplished had you been the striped feline's latest conquest.

There was an English professor in college that I absolutely couldn't stand. He was the only one who taught a class that was required for my major. It drove me bonkers to go to his class every day, but I knew if I wanted to graduate with my chosen major, I would have to take his class. Begrudgingly, I attended class the entire semester because I knew it was necessary to accomplish my goal of graduating. In hindsight, however, I could have shifted my attitude!

Both of these stories clearly demonstrate a sense of motivation. Motivation is having a carrot in front of you or a tiger behind. Either one may get you to move, but they are both external.

Motivation and inspiration are often used interchangeably; however, there is one major difference. When the external motivation disappears, we often come to a screeching halt. With inspiration, the internal factors that cause us to act are lasting.

Certainly, there are times we decide to do or not do something because we are motivated. Personally, I can't stand working with numbers. I recognize, however, that there are certain times in my life when I will have to deal with numbers. I am motivated to do so because I want to know what is in the bank account.

I can also shift my focus from knowing the numbers in the bank account to thinking about what it is that I would love to do with my money. What gifts would I give? What vacations would I take? What improvements might I make to my home?

Those things inspire me. Not only is it much easier to focus on the task at hand, but it gives me a sense of purpose as I do it.

You may not feel inspired to go to the gym and workout, but do you feel inspired to teach your children healthy habits? It may not feel inspiring to run on a treadmill, but maybe hiking in the nearby mountains does.

Act from inspiration rather than motivation. When your actions are inspired, they will have a lasting effect on your habitual way of being.

Motivation can also play an important role as you are beginning your journey. It may be difficult to make any correlation between your actions and what inspires you. Find a place where you are able to recognize whether you are acting from motivation or inspiration. If you realize your actions are motivated, see if you can find something that also inspires you to act in the same way.

Chapter Ten Lessons:

- Motivation is having a carrot in front of you or a tiger behind.

- With inspiration, the internal factors that cause us to act are lasting.

- Act from inspiration rather than motivation. When your actions are inspired, they will have a lasting effect on your habitual way of being.

- If you realize your actions are motivated, see if you can find something that also inspires you to act in the same way.

Chapter Ten Affirmation:

"I choose to turn my motivations into inspiration so that my actions have a lasting effect on my habitual way of being. I find people, emotions, and things that provide inspiration to act in a way that is healthy for both myself and the universe around me. Today, I choose inspiration."

Chapter Eleven:
Someone to Watch Over Me

We all need someone to be our cheerleader, our fellow traveler, and our inspiration. We also need someone to tell us when we have food in our teeth, when we've really screwed up, and when we need to get it together. Your Fitness Friend is just that.

I highly recommend that on your journey, you find someone whom you can talk to at least once a week. I usually do **not** suggest that this person be a significant other, spouse, family member, or even close friend unless you feel you are able to be business-like and completely honest with each other.

The purpose of a Fitness Friend is not really to have a "buddy," but to ensure you are following through with your commitments. They may enforce motivating consequences if you do not follow through. Often times, a Fitness Friend can become a very close friend through the process. No matter your relationship, try to focus on the goals at hand.

You can meet as often as every day and it can be done in person or over the phone. Here are some guidelines:

1. Set up a regular meeting time.
2. Begin with what's "new and good"
3. Decide who will begin.
4. Respect your partner's time.
5. Keep the length of the call at least 10 minutes but no longer than 1 hour.
6. Discuss your current challenges.
7. Listen to feedback.
8. Set motivational consequences.

9. Create action steps to be completed by the next meeting.
10. Take notes and review them. (optional)

A good Fitness Friend will listen to your challenges, celebrate your successes, and let you know when you are falling short of your commitments. They are not there to commiserate with you or help you feel sorry for yourself. Your conversations may not always feel comfortable. You may be challenged. Remember, it's not comfortable to be told when you have food in your teeth, but think about how grateful you are once they tell you!

Once you have set up a time and frequency to meet, you will both get the chance to celebrate any successes for a few moments. This can be anything from a simple, "I skipped the fast food yesterday" to "I have accomplished my 6-month goal in only 4 months!" Keep this short, but really celebrate any accomplishments, insights, or "aha's."

You'll want to give each other equal time to share your current challenge. Make sure to leave ample time for your Fitness Friend to offer solutions. Before ending the conversation, you'll want to set a goal to accomplish before your next meeting. It should be a little bit of a stretch. The point is to get you to do something more than you might normally do. If you or your Fitness Friend has doubts about your commitment to the goal, you'll want to set some motivational consequences. For example, if you are someone who loves to wear fur, you might really hate to write a check to PETA. As a consequence if you choose not to follow through with your commitment, your Fitness Friend might suggest you write a substantial check to PETA.

Once you both agree on a motivational consequence, you will both reiterate your commitments for your next meeting and, if you like, memorialize them in a note or e-mail so as not to forget. Now that someone else is aware of your commitment, it makes it that much more difficult to back out (especially if you have to write a check you really don't want to write!).

If you do become great friends (or if you already were) with your Fitness Friend, make sure you do not slip into chit-chat. You might wish to schedule additional time during your meeting for chatting, but make sure to keep the structure of the meeting during the actual meeting time.

You may find that it works out to work out with your Fitness Friend, but it's ok to have a Fitness Friend and a workout buddy. You will want to build a support system with few, if any, holes in it. The more people you get on your team, the easier your success will seem.

Along with your Fitness Friend, think of other supporters you may be able to add to your team. Maybe your family would like to join you and get fit, maybe your coworkers would love to be held accountable at lunch, and maybe you would like to hire a personal trainer or nutritionist.

Let others know your goals and how they can support you. You will be surprised at all the opportunities that spring up as you just ask for the support you need. It is human nature to want to help each other.

Chapter Eleven Lessons:

- ➢ Your Fitness Friend is someone who will tell you when you have food in your teeth.

- ➢ The purpose of a Fitness Friend is not really to have a "buddy," but to ensure you are following through with your commitments.

- ➢ Along with your Fitness Friend, think of other supporters you may be able to add to your team.

- ➢ Let others know your goals and let them know how they can support you.

Chapter Eleven Affirmation:

"I build a team to help support me in the accomplishment of my goals. My Fitness Friend helps hold me accountable in the times of challenge. My team builds me up and serves as a gentle reminder of my life purpose. My team also consists of all those who have gone on similar journeys before me as their wisdom is easily accessible in the universe which surrounds me. I have a great team!"

Chapter Twelve:
Cavemen Did It

I am not the first to tell you all that fad diets do not work. You may lose weight by eating only grapefruit for a week or doing a juice fast; however, there are serious nutritional deficiencies that after some time may begin to affect you negatively.

The human race has become so disconnected from nature that we often forget that we are part of the animal kingdom. For eons, the diet of most animals has remained the same. The animal kingdom has also remained relatively healthy, unless those animals happen to be in captivity. Do you see any overweight lions walking around? How about huge increases in diabetes or cancer within the elephant population? These animals have continued to eat innately and have therefore been able to thrive from a nutritional standpoint.

It stands to reason that if animals are eating the same diet they have for thousands of years and have remained healthy, we might do well to follow their lead on this one. It is estimated that the human genetic code has changed only about .02% since the beginning of man. Our diet, however, has been dramatically altered.

Paleolithic man ate a diet consisting primarily of vegetables, fruit, and lean protein. It's that simple. Much of this was consumed raw, which maintains the integrity of absorbable nutrients in the food.

So, what does this mean for you, a human being living in today's world of hamburgers, French fries, and chocolate shakes? Let me start by setting your mind at ease a bit. I am by no means perfect when it comes to my diet. I love the flavor of coffee, I have been known to indulge in an ice cream, and I have eaten my share of burgers and fries. Eating according to the Paleolithic diet is not a make or break "diet," but rather a lifestyle, a new way of looking at food, and a guideline.

Most everyone knows what a vegetable is. Most of us know we should eat more of them; however, the number one consumed vegetable in the U.S. has consistently been the potato…French-fried. Many of our typical meals contain few, if any vegetables.

If you are one of the folks who used to slip your broccoli to the dog (as my dad still does), it's time to be a grown-up and at least try your veggies.

Many of us are better about fruit, simply because we love that sweet factor. Fruit is best eaten by itself simply because it is digested so quickly; however, I am not a stickler and I do not hold anyone to a higher standard than I keep myself.

On a bit of a side note, grocery store vegetables have done nothing for the popularity of the vegetable (or fruit for that matter) as the vast majority are picked long before ripe, shipped across countries, and sit on the shelf for substantial amounts of time. Grocery stores have also chosen certain varieties of vegetables because of their uniform look or potential shelf life. This means that taste is often not top on the considerations list. Having eaten from my local farmer's markets and organic family farms for several years, I may seem a bit of a fruit/veggie snob, but it truly tastes better! I have also been exposed to myriad varieties that have become new favorites and I look forward to their seasons!

Many of us have no idea what is in season in our area at any particular time of year because we have grown so accustomed to finding tomatoes, potatoes, broccoli, and apples whenever we feel like eating one. Eating fresh fruit and vegetables that are in season is

Mind Over Fatter: The Secret to Thinking Yourself Thin

a wholly different experience from eating the cardboard apples or the less-than-sweet strawberries found year-round.

Nuts and seeds are also part of the Paleolithic man's diet; however be aware of the processing that goes on with some of these. Virtually all peanuts and peanut butter also contain a carcinogenic substance called aflatoxin, so I tend to avoid them unless they are organic (though this does not guarantee aflatoxin isn't present, it greatly reduces the probability). For the sake of fairness, many other grains and nuts can contain aflatoxins, but peanut butter is the most common.

If you live in the United States, you have no doubt been taught or at least shown some form of the Food Guide Pyramid. Prominently displayed at the foundation of the pyramid or in the largest section of the most recent version, you will find the grains/bread/cereal category.

I believe this is a gross misrepresentation of the nutritional needs of the human being. But, don't believe a word I say. I am not a doctor. I encourage you to do your own, independent research.

It is estimated that at least one in every three people is gluten-intolerant. Gluten is the protein found in wheat, barley, and rye. The gluten molecule is too large to be digested by human beings and can cause myriad ailments. When I say gluten-intolerant, I am not referring to celiac disease (though celiac disease is one type of gluten intolerance). It is highly possible to be intolerant to gluten, yet not have celiac. Celiac disease affects the intestinal tract; however, gluten can affect many other organs and can be the cause of many other symptoms, including depression, fatigue, arthritis, constipation, diarrhea, and aches and pains.

In my case, gluten was seriously affecting my adrenal glands and was causing fatigue and depression. Seeking a natural approach, I had tried homeopathy, herbs, eliminating meat and dairy, and chiropractic. While these were all very helpful, my system could not withstand a daily onslaught of something I was highly allergic to.

The best news is that it will not cost you anything to find out if you are gluten intolerant. All you have to do is eliminate it from your diet to find out if it is affecting you. Gluten can be found in many things other than your typical bread, cereals, and flour-based products. Soy sauce, soups, beer, herbal teas (in the form of barley malt), and even some ice creams are some of the most common offenders.

To learn more about gluten intolerance and celiac disease, check out *Life After Bread* by Dr. Eydi Bauer, D.C. It is a quick read with some great references to get you on the right track immediately.

Lean protein refers to any meat, poultry, or fish that is prepared without a large amount of oil or fat. Be mindful of the fact that Paleolithic man would find and kill a wild animal and eat it over a period of time. Today, we "raise" meat, poultry, and fish, and pollute our environment. We also feed our animals food that is not on their innate meal plan, so they may not be healthy either. I will go into that in more detail in a later chapter.

Again, if you were looking for a "diet" or strict meal plan, I am sorry to disappoint. The Paleolithic diet is very simple in nature, but can still be excellent when it comes to your taste buds. Ultimately, it is up to you to find something that works for you. I will tell you that I have seen countless numbers of people have much success eating this way, and I know it works.

As with any lifestyle change, it works best to control your environment at least for a while, which is why it may behoove you to learn to cook or prepare some easy meals at home. This may be the perfect opportunity to learn to cook, or to enhance your skills!

Mind Over Fatter: The Secret to Thinking Yourself Thin

It may help you to create "policies" for your eating lifestyle if you are someone who thrives in a more structured environment. These could look something like this:

1. I will restrict eating gluten to a piece of cake on my actual birthday.
2. I buy only "clean" meat (organic and free from hormones, antibiotics, etc.)
3. I eat all the vegetables on my plate before tasting anything else.

Pick the policies that work for you. These policies can not only serve as a guideline for you, but also help you explain your position to others without feeling as if you have offended them by not partaking in their home-baked bread or having a bite of turkey before trying the veggies.

Chapter Twelve Lessons:

- Fad diets do not work.

- It is estimated that the human genetic code has changed only about .02% since the beginning of man. Our diet, however, has been dramatically altered.

- Paleolithic man ate a diet consisting primarily of vegetables, fruit, and lean protein.

- Create "policies" for your eating lifestyle if you are someone who thrives in a more structured environment.

Chapter Twelve Affirmation:

"My diet nourishes and supports my physical body. I make choices that assist me in fulfillment of my purpose and I create policies to serve as guidelines to keep me on track."

Chapter Thirteen:
Conscious Consumers

On a ride on the Amtrak down the California coast, one might see plenty of cattle grazing upon open, green fields. Calves jump and frolic with one another as their maternal counterparts seem blissfully unaware of the dangers that may befall their young. The vast amount of green along the California shoreline is a strange juxtaposition of ranchers and beach bums; however, it is reminiscent of a much simpler time. A time when people raised their own cattle and chickens, ate vegetables from their own plot of land, and even churned their own butter.

While there are times I get lost in this dreamy-eyed version of "simple," I am not so naïve to think that this is the dream of many. Perhaps it may even be your own personal nightmare! There is, however, much to be said for creating awareness about where your food comes from.

What type of world do you wish to live in? Does your ideal world consist of a peaceful, loving community for all concerned, including the cattle we raise for slaughter? If so, then where is your disconnect?

As a society, we have completely forgotten the origin of our food and as a result have become numb (or ignorant) to the way it is processed. Very few thank the cow when we sit down for our Mickey D's. No ceremony is required, but once you begin to really think consciously about what you are putting into your mouth, you may find that what you put into your mouth begins to change.

Not all who read this book will decide to become strict locavores (those who eat only locally produced food grown sustainably and organically) and be completely mindful about where their food comes from. We have already addressed pesticides, herbicides, organic, and hormones and I will not belabor that point.

Many of us have dogs, cats, birds, bunnies, horses, reptiles, etc., whom we consider part of our family and the thought of someone slaughtering our "babies" to eat them would churn our stomach. So why should it be any different for our animal friends whom we have decided to consider food?

Though I have been a vegetarian for some relatively brief periods in my life, it is not something I typically recommend from a health perspective. Many vegetarians, however, are people who began researching the way we treat our animals and have made an ethical choice not to consume them. But that is not the goal of this chapter.

Think about where your food comes from. If you're not sure, ask. Read some books or articles or watch some films about what exactly happens to the animals we consider food. You may find that the choices you make are much different.

As much as we hate to think about it, we are part of the animal kingdom. Humans are animals. Would we resort to cannibalism should survival become a factor? Maybe. Would we decide to eat each other just because we thought we tasted good? The answer for the vast majority of us would probably be in the negative. Even worse, if we did decide we liked the taste of human flesh, would we mass produce it and treat each other with complete disrespect and cruelty? I personally would not want to live in that world regardless of which side of the coin I was on. Is this all sounding a bit morbid or soilent-green-ish to you? It should.

Health comes from within, but this is only possible if we have the ability to give ourselves quality fuel and a safe environment. Given the current state of our food economy, neither of these will be possible in a very short period of time.

Mind Over Fatter: The Secret to Thinking Yourself Thin

So, why be a conscious consumer? Contrary to popular belief, it is not for me to build my free-loving, hippie commune. Conscious consumption of food should concern each and every one of us and our subsequent generations.

Here is how the cycle works:

Rancher is not making substantial income to support his family and decides to industrialize his operation.

Rancher sells some land or gets some outside (usually corporate) funding to purchase additional heads of cattle.

Corporate consumers (ultimately, the cheeseburger-consuming public) begin pushing for more production.

Rancher tries to produce by placing more cattle on the same plot of land. Corporate consumers ask for more product and demand it more quickly.

Rancher feeds cattle corn and other byproducts and administers growth hormones to fatten them up at a quicker pace.

Corporate food pushes more hamburgers, bigger patties, additional patties, 2-for-1 deals, etc., and the demand increases.

Repeat cycle...over and over and over.

So, who is really winning here? The end-result is that consumers (or the burger eaters) are becoming sick, overweight, and unhealthy. The ranchers are often not making enough money to sustain their families. The corporate big wigs, well...who knows? All the money in the world cannot buy happiness, but maybe if they stay away from the very product they are hawking, they at least have a chance at health. Harsh? Maybe. Honest? Definitely.

Let me expand a bit on what happens to the planet during all of this. You may not have any desire to become a card-carrying member of The Sierra Club or the green movement but the fact is that we do have ONE environment in which we live and currently, that environment is called Earth. On an even larger scale, that environment is called the Universe. Remember also, that we are now taking 100% responsibility for our lives. That most definitely includes how we are contributing to the destruction of our environment.

In the case of cattle, they are often enclosed in very tight pens and are fed a substantial amount of food. As a side note, cattle are not meant to eat corn, feed, or anything else besides grass. I have seen cattle grazing upon potato chips and M&M's, believe it or not. Cattle are a multi-stomached, ruminant animal, which means they are designed to eat grass. What happens when you eat something you know you are not designed to eat?

Well, the same thing happens to cattle. They get sick. Much of that "sickness" comes out their rear end and they wallow in it until someone comes along and moves it to a large manure lagoon where it festers, leeches into ground water, or makes its way down to the ocean. You may ask, "Well, isn't that what normally happens?" Actually, no. In a large field where cattle are free to graze (and poop) on the grass, the manure is graciously spread out and acts as a natural fertilizer. In fact, many true organic farmers will rotate their animals and bring the chickens into the pasture a couple days after the cattle to pick out the maggot larvae (which they love) and consequently, distribute the manure throughout the land. It is tremendously efficient and the perfect example of Mother Nature working in harmony. It is only when the manure is highly concentrated that it becomes a problem.

The cattle, however, also become sick in many other capacities. Ranchers then take a proactive approach and vaccinate their cattle, administer antibiotics, and feed medicated feed which serves to further contaminate the end-product and makes for an even more uncomfortable, unbearable life for our four-legged counterparts.

Keep in mind, this is not meant to scare you into vegetarianism, but to make you think about what you are eating and where it comes from. If you are interested in learning more about this topic, pick up *The Omnivore's Dilemma* or *In Defense of Food* both by Michael Pollan.

Conscious food consumers not only create better physical health for themselves simply because they choose to eat a much higher quality of food, but they contribute to the health of our environment, which, in turn, benefits us all. Eat consciously!

Chapter Thirteen Lessons:

- Once you begin to really think consciously about what you are putting into your mouth, you may find that what you put into your mouth begins to change.

- Health comes from within, but this is only possible if we have the ability to give ourselves quality fuel and a safe environment. Given the current state of our food economy, neither of these will be possible in a very short period of time.

- Conscious food consumers not only create better physical health for themselves simply because they choose to eat a much higher quality of food, but they contribute to the health of our environment, which, in turn, benefits us all.

Chapter Thirteen Affirmation:

"I choose to eat consciously. In doing so, I know that I am benefitting my body and the planet. Because of my conscious choices, future generations will be able to consume healthy food. I am a conscious consumer."

Chapter Fourteen:
You Like to Move It!

OK, let's face it. In order to accomplish your health and fitness goals, you are going to have to make a commitment to move. Movement is life. Movement is health. We are called "animate," which plainly means we move. Anything "inanimate" does not move, and therefore, is not alive. The more you lean towards inanimate, the closer you flirt with the idea of death. This may seem harsh or scary, but it is the truth.

I know, I know. Many of you were dreading this chapter. Some of you were looking forward to getting a clear-cut answer about what exercise program is the best. I have to apologize because I do not have an answer to that question. The great news is that YOU DO!

Take out your journal or a piece of paper and make a list of 25 things you absolutely love to do. When you do these things, time seems to stand still and you could do them all day. Don't worry about making this about exercise. It's not. Write down the things you truly love to do.

I asked a friend to make a list and the following is what she came up with:

1. **Have great conversation with my son**
2. **Connect with positive and inspiring people**
3. **Learn, learn, learn**
4. **Stroll on the beach**
5. Snuggle with my doggie
6. Take naps

7. Any and all spa treatments
8. Educate and inspire others to find peace, joy, and harmony
9. **Travel**
10. **Sleep**
11. Eat out
12. **Mentor with Jack Canfield**
13. Attend Agape Center services
14. Get my make-up and hair done
15. **See my family and friends happy**
16. **Volunteer**
17. Attend Musicals
18. **Go to Museums**
19. **See Jon Bon Jovi in concert**
20. **Shop**
21. Eat Ice Cream
22. Listen to the ocean
23. **Laugh**
24. **Be my authentic self**
25. Hold and cuddle babies

I have bolded 14 out of her 25 things because all of these things she can do while she is exercising. She may wish to stroll on the beach with her son (or even talk to him on the phone while she is doing it). She could travel to Italy and walk much of her time there. Sleep is an integral component of health, so that will contribute to her success even though it does not involve moving. Jack Canfield always has yoga and kickboxing classes offered before each of his longer workshops, and she could certainly connect with positive, inspiring people while she was there. She could volunteer planting trees or playing with children, dance her heart out at Bon Jovi concerts, walk the mall or museum a few times, laughing burns calories, and she could be her authentic self no matter what she was doing.

Mind Over Fatter: The Secret to Thinking Yourself Thin

The point is that you can incorporate exercise into everything you love to do. It doesn't have to be a chore or something you dread. Chances are if you dread it, you won't do it!

Look at your list and see how many you may be able to do while exercising. Some of your loves may actually be something active. How can you do those things more often? If it's dancing, join a dance class. If it's swimming, find a body of water (and maybe buy a wetsuit!). If it's hiking, find a trail you like and schedule it in your day. Not only will you find that exercise becomes easy, but you will be doing things you love to do!

This may seem a bit too simple for some of you. That's because it is. No crazy contraptions, no expensive memberships, no outrageous promises. Do what you love and the fitness will follow.

Certainly, there are several things I have done and enjoyed, and I am happy to share my experience with them; however, it would only be my experience. Your experience with dance class may be completely different than mine. I have always been active, but sports weren't really my thing. And believe it or not, I still am not a big fan of running.

You don't need to be an athlete or a yogi master or an expert to move your body and get exercise. You just need to have a body and have the ability to move it.

Chapter Fourteen Lessons:

- In order to accomplish your health and fitness goals, you are going to have to make a commitment to move.

- You can incorporate exercise into everything you love to do.

- Do what you love and the fitness will follow.

- You don't need to be an athlete or a yogi master or an expert to move your body and get exercise. You just need to have a body and have the ability to move it.

Chapter Fourteen Affirmation:

"I choose to keep my body active doing things I love to do. Movement is not only effortless, but fun! I am grateful for the ability to move my body and to show my gratitude, I move it!"

Chapter Fifteen:
Committed

We have all made a commitment at some point in our lives. Often, when we think of commitment, we immediately think of our commitments to others. Making a commitment to get fit and healthy is a commitment to you. If you fall off the treadmill and you don't get back on, most likely, the only one who seems disappointed is you.

Unfortunately, it is often your commitments to you that get put on the back burner or pushed out another day. Have you ever listened to the airline stewards remind you that in case of an emergency, you should always put on your mask first? You can never be any help to others if you don't take care of you!

Staying committed to your health and fitness goals will not only help you become a better you, but a better mother, father, sister, brother, son, daughter, boss, employee, friend, or spouse. Your commitment to yourself means so much to so many other people who depend upon you.

Staying committed simply means taking everything one day at a time, one stair step at a time, and one choice at a time. You will learn what helps you and what hinders you. You will learn where you excel and where you struggle. You will learn when you need support and when you feel autonomous.

You can only do your best with all the tools and knowledge you have at this moment. Tomorrow, you may know more. Tomorrow, you may weigh less. Tomorrow, you may take a fall.

Your commitment to yourself is the most crucial commitment you can make because it is from that commitment that all the others stem. Your commitment to your health and fitness is the foundation for everything else.

Anyone who ever succeeded at anything made the commitment to do so. Do you think Steve Jobs or Richard Branson decided to form their respective businesses without committing wholly to the concept? The amount of their success depended upon their commitment to make it happen.

You can exercise the same kind of dedication to your commitment as the most successful entrepreneurs in business, the most successful married couples, or the most successful parents on the planet did when they set out to create success.

Love does not have to mean self-sacrificing behavior. Remember that in order to fully love others, you must fully love yourself first! And we tend to take good care of those we love! Love who you are in the moment and make a commitment to show yourself love by making choices that support your commitment!

Chapter Fifteen Lessons:

- Making a commitment to get fit and healthy, however, is a commitment to you.

- Your commitment to yourself means so much to so many other people who depend upon you.

- You can only do your best with all the tools and knowledge you have at this moment.

- Your commitment to yourself is the most crucial commitment you can make because it is from that commitment that all the others stem. Your commitment to your health and fitness is the foundation for everything else.

Chapter Fifteen Affirmation:

"I choose today to make a commitment to myself. Committing to my health and fitness means I am saying 'yes' to me. Others depend on me to be the best I can be and I can only do so when I am feeling my best. I am committed to me."

Chapter Sixteen:
Falling Off the Treadmill

I love the synergy of group classes at the gym and so I tend to schedule my exercise by choosing a group class to attend. One particular day, I walked into the gym without any prior knowledge of the class schedule and saw they were just about to start an advanced step class. I was confident that with my dance background and excellent coordination, the class would be a breeze. I proceeded to grab a step and not one, but two sets of risers. (For those of you unfamiliar with step classes, risers are the little squares you but under the step to make it higher.)

Class began and through the warm-up, I kept up to speed (almost). As we progressed into the first combination, however, I quickly realized I was in way over my head. The instructor called out move after move and I found myself utterly unfamiliar with the step lingo. "Around the world, Over the top, Straddle down, V-step..." she said. Before long, I found myself watching her every move and totally determined to get it right. As I continued my futile effort to catch on, she promptly changed the combination. I watched her expertly execute the new move and simultaneously attempted to do it and that's when things went awry. I somehow missed the step, kicked it off the risers, and fell to my knees. Yes, I completely fell. To make matters worse, the instructor immediately stopped teaching to make sure I was ok. I was just fine, thank you, but I was ready to call it a day.

Inevitably there will be times when you too will fall off your step. The falling is actually not the problem at all. It is truly the getting back up that really counts. When you fall off that treadmill, remember that you are not alone. I do not know of anyone who has not fallen at least once.

Your fall may be like mine, quite literal. It may also be more of an emotional fall such as one might experience when a relationship is in turmoil or you lose your job. No matter the reason for the fall, remember your purpose, your goals, and your desires. Nobody else can make the decision to get back up. You can certainly ask for a hand to reach down and help you up, but ultimately, the decision lies in your hands.

I did decide that step aerobics might not be the ideal class for me, but I have taken a few classes since then. Despite my bruised ankle (ahem…read ego), I went back to the gym the very next day.

Prepare yourself for a few slips off the treadmill along the way. Most importantly, when it happens, stop the treadmill, take a deep breath, and get back on.

Chapter Sixteen Lessons:

- Inevitably there will be times when you too will fall off the treadmill.

- Your fall may be quite literal or it may also be more of an emotional fall such as one might experience when a relationship is in turmoil or you lose your job.

- Nobody else can make the decision to get back up. You can certainly ask for a hand to reach down and help you up, but ultimately, the decision lies in your hands.

- Prepare yourself for a few slips off the treadmill along the way. Most importantly, when it happens, stop the treadmill, take a deep breath, and get back on.

Chapter Sixteen Affirmation:

"Though I may fall off my treadmill, I know that I can get back on. My strength allows me to get back on and keep going. I choose to persevere with my goals in mind. I choose to get back on the treadmill."

Chapter Seventeen:
Oh, What Fun!

Recently, while having breakfast with a friend I stated, "Well, we're all here to learn!"

He shocked me by responding, "No we're not!" I must say I was initially taken aback. I thought; *what does he know that I don't?*

He laughed as I tend to wear my emotions on my face and said, "We're all here to have fun!"

"Ah…" I said. That sounded much better!

Life really is all about having fun. We are given such a very short time on this earth that it would be a shame to feel like you had "worked" your entire life.

My point is very simple. Whether you are riding jet skis, having a party, travelling, exercising, or eating healthy, it should be fun! The goal of this book is not to make everything seem like a struggle, but to allow you to feel your healthiest and have fun doing it.

We have talked about incorporating exercise and movement into something you love to do, but I often hear it is the nutrition piece that feels slightly less "fun." Many feel they must "give up" things they enjoy or trade their French fries in for their…green salad?!

There are so many wonderful resources for people who are looking for healthy (and tasty!) options that you might find yourself more than pleasantly surprised. If cooking is a little too daunting for you at first, you may want to check your area for restaurants that offer organic, vegan, vegetarian, gluten-free, or even raw options. Several raw restaurants are sprouting up all over that serve delicious and filling meals. Play detective and see what you come up with! If the options are not obvious, try asking at your local gym or friends that seem to eat more healthfully.

You can also seek these places out when you travel. You may be amazed at how good healthy food can look and taste.

As an avid cook, I found it inspiring to discover and create new recipes. I felt like the Julia Child of healthy cooking as I encountered new ingredients and new ways to prepare old stand-bys.

When my local CSA (Community Supported Agriculture) basket arrived each week, it felt like Christmas. What would I get this week? How could I put things together? What the heck is a parsnip? Not every culinary feat was deemed a success, but it certainly was a blast preparing it!

I learned to make homemade non-dairy ice cream, raw, vegan truffles, vegetable casseroles, and kale salads. My kitchen was a disaster, but I subscribe to the "It's more fun making the mess" club anyway.

If you enjoy shopping, maybe it will be the healthy gourmet foods, seeking out new dinner plates that are smaller in size, or buying new (smaller!) clothes that become fun for you. Maybe it will be the chance to get together for potlucks with friends who are on the same path or the opportunity to run the community 5k.

I have always thought the term "working out" was not only a misnomer, but also a funny way to refer to something that could be fun. I mean, who wants to "work out?" I would much rather go out dancing, go for a nature hike, swim in the pool, snorkel, or learn how to surf. That sounds like fun!

Mind Over Fatter: The Secret to Thinking Yourself Thin

Though I also happened to enjoy yoga classes and weight lifting, it is because I enjoy it that I go back. We are all familiar with the crowds in the gym come January 1 each year. It's no wonder they are back to square one by March. Everybody joins because they make a resolution that this will be the year they get healthy. So, they jump on the treadmill, lift weights, and take a class or two. But sooner or later it stops being fun and they stop going.

It's not that their intentions weren't there, but that they chose to do an activity they did not find fun or exciting. Their motivation might have kept them going for a while, but after the motivation faded, they realized they were not inspired to keep going back.

My recommendation is this: If any of this ceases being fun, stop and rethink your approach. Accomplishing lasting results relies upon it.

Chapter Seventeen Lessons:

- Life really is all about having fun.

- You don't have to "give up" anything if you look at all the things you stand to gain.

- Stop "working out" and start having fun.

- If any of this ceases being fun, stop and rethink your approach. Accomplishing lasting results relies upon it.

Chapter Seventeen Affirmation:

"I choose today to have fun! I find joy in each new adventure as I make my way toward health and fitness. I no longer 'work out'; I have fun! In fact, I am so busy having fun that attaining my results becomes easy and effortless. I choose today to have FUN!"

Epilogue

This book is truly the result of the many tools I thought people were asking for when they approached me about losing weight. It wasn't until I conquered my own battle with weight that I truly understood what others like me were in need of.

You see, I gave people all the tools necessary to succeed. I would map out a nutrition plan, a fitness plan, set some goals, and even hold them accountable. I thought that maybe if I gave my clients better tools or more information, they would succeed. As a result, I devoured every book I could get my hands on and listened to every speech or interview I could find. Though I could answer all the questions my clients were asking, I couldn't answer the ones they weren't.

When they didn't show for class, told me they slipped up on their nutrition, or quit the program altogether, I thought it must have been something I wasn't doing right. It was. But not in the way I thought. I could get them to change their nutrition and fitness habits with no problem, but I couldn't change the way they looked at themselves.

When I talk with someone who calls themselves a "yo-yo dieter", or big boned, or fat and happy, I don't give them tools anymore. It's not the tools that are important.

The journey to health and fitness does not lie in some magic pill or special diet or even in your genes. It lies within your mind.

Am I saying that simply changing your mind-set will change your health and fitness? Not entirely. There are definitely tools involved. What I am saying is that the tools only become effective once you address the thoughts, the emotions, and the self-images that are holding you back.

Have I fallen off the treadmill throughout my journey? Of course. Will I do it again? Probably. I don't take myself so seriously that I lose sight of the forest for the trees. You just might catch me doing something I have talked about not doing. Nothing is absolute.

My wish for you is that you treat yourself, and therefore your physical body, with the love and respect it deserves. You are too valuable to shorten your life by making poor choices. Have you ever been saddened to see someone else not living up to their potential? There are so many people that depend upon the fulfillment of your purpose.

I love you. I am grateful for you. May you find innumerable blessings on your journey to health and happiness and as always, have FUN!

Love & Gratitude~

Erin

Mind Over Fatter
Recommended Resources

For Mind Over Fatter workshops, keynotes and teleseminars, and camps presented by Erin Tullius

Visit www.MindOverFatterBook.com

The following is a partial list of books, workshops, films and audio programs which inspired the writing of this book:

The Success Principles: How to Get From Where You Are To Where You Want to Be, by Jack Canfield with Janet Switzer

The Secret, film by Rhonda Byrne

Breakthrough to Success, audio program by Jack Canfield

Canfield Training Group "Breakthrough to Success" week-long intensive, "Advanced Training" program, and year-long "Train the Trainer" program

The Innate Diet & Natural Hygiene, by Dr. James Chestnut

The Biology of Belief, by Dr. Bruce Lipton

Success in General:

The Power of Focus: How to Hit Your Business, Personal, and Financial Targets with Absolute Certainty, by Jack Canfield, Mark Victor Hansen, and Les Hewitt

Think and Grow Rich, By Napoleon Hill

Unlimited Power, By Anthony Robbins

Ask and It is Given: Learning to Manifest Your Desires, by Esther and Jerry Hicks

Inspiration and Motivation

Chicken Soup for the Soul, series by Jack Canfield and Mark Victor Hansen

It's Not Over Until You Win, by Les Brown

Personal Development, Inner Peace and Spirituality

The Sedona Method: Your Key to Lasting Happiness, Success, and Emotional Well-being, by Hale Dwoskin

The Four Agreements: A Practical Guide to Personal Freedom, by Don Miguel Ruiz

Power vs. Force: The Hidden Dimension of Human Behavior, by David R. Hawkins

The Power of Now: A Guide to Spiritual Enlightenment, by Eckhart Tolle

The Way of the Peaceful Warrior, by Dan Millman (also a film)

A New Earth: Awakening to Your Life's Purpose, by Eckhart Tolle

Human Potential Trainings

Canfield Training Group, www.canfieldtrainings.com or www.jackcanfield.com
Phone: 805-563-2935. Programs throughout the world from 1-day to year-long programs.

Landmark Education (Landmark Forum), www.landmarkeducation.com, Phone: 415-981-8850. A weekend seminar to take you out of fear and into living a dynamic, intentional life. Expect greater self-esteem, more fulfilling relationships, greater financial success, and more balance in your life.

Sedona Training Associates, www.sedona.com, Phone: 928-282-3522. One of the easiest and most powerful methods for releasing emotions, fears, anxieties, anger, depression, and finding lasting peace, joy, and love.

Health and Wellness

www.shakeology.com/mindoverfatter
To purchase Shakeology (the superfood meal-replacement shake Erin recommends)

www.beachbodycoach.com/mindoverfatter
Find out more about P90X, Insanity, Turbo Jam, Hip Hop Abs and many other Beachbody programs (the at-home fitness programs recommended by Erin)

The Innate Series, books by Dr. James Chestnut. Trainings also available. www.thewellnesspractice.com

JJ Virgin and Associates. Web-based program featuring nutritional counseling, products, and ideal menus and recipes. www.jjvirgin.com

Life After Bread by Dr. Eydi Bauer- An excellent, informative, and quick read on gluten-intolerance and Celiac disease

About the Author

Erin Tullius is a pioneer in both the human potential and wellness fields and is in demand as a heartfelt speaker. An avid student of natural living practices, Erin is passionate about communicating and sharing her experience of personal growth coupled with a naturally healthy lifestyle.

Erin is a certified Pilates instructor, and has been described as a wellness coach and motivator wrapped into one. She has studied with Dr. James Chestnut and immersed herself in the works of Michael Pollan and others of like mind. She was accepted and graduated from her personal mentor, Jack Canfield's inaugural Train the Trainer program in 2010 and studies human potential with a voracious curiosity. This is her first book.

Erin, age 30, is a graduate of Chapman University and now resides on the Central Coast of California with her husband Steve and young son Tyler.

LaVergne, TN USA
23 October 2010
201958LV00004B/1/P